MW01717218

15% WRONG

The Outrageous Truth About Medical Misdiagnosis

by

Dr. Richard Griffith, D.Engr. Sci., M.D.

Author
Dr. Richard Griffith, Guilford, VT
Publisher
Dr. Russ Hill, Laguna Beach, CA
Editor
Dr. Art Dimock, Woodstock Valley, CT

Introduction

Leslie was 48 years old, married, with three children. She smoked cigarettes but was trying to end that unhealthy habit. Smoking started in college, perhaps proving to herself that she had become an adult and could make such decisions. But now, several decades later, Leslie regretted that decision.

It had been a tough week at her job, but she needed to work to ensure the family could afford college tuition for the kids. They were growing up almost too fast, it seemed. Early in the week, she had vague stomach pains that radiated into her lower back. The pain nagged but had ebbed by mid-week. But late Friday afternoon, the ache returned with a vengeance. She made it through dinner but finally asked her husband to take her to the hospital to be on the safe side.

They were fortunate to have a great hospital in their community near the coast of Maryland. It was part of a statewide sophisticated trauma network that Maryland had pioneered. At the Emergency Room, she was promptly evaluated and, within 30 minutes, had the full attention of a senior general surgeon who was an officer of the Medical Staff and highly respected throughout the community.

In medical school, students learn that gallbladder disease occurs most commonly in females with four specific characteristics, each starting with the letter F: Fair, Fat, Flocculent, and Forty. Flocculent may seem confusing. The dictionary says flocculent means resembling tufts of wool. Perhaps when scholars originally coined the Four-Fs to define the nature of gallbladder disease, that word had a more widely appreciated meaning. Or, maybe adding that word made the concept more memorable for those who needed to salt it away permanently in their memory bank. In any case, Leslie fit the criteria with all the proper symptoms. Plus, pressing on her abdomen elicited the responses the surgeon was expecting to verify his diagnosis.

It still made sense to get additional confirmation, so an attendant wheeled Leslie away to the radiology suite for an ultrasound examination of her gallbladder. Sure enough, she had gallstones, tiny globs of solidified digestive juices that looked like ten pieces of driveway gravel inside the three-inch long narrow gallbladder sac tucked up under the front edge of the liver. That confirmed the diagnosis, and Leslie soon headed off to surgery. It was not an immediate emergency, but an operating room was available and fully staffed with no reason not to perform surgery that would quickly get her back to good health.

We need to add more information about gallbladder disease to make sense of this situation. Gallbladder pain occurs because gallstones eventually grow large enough to no longer pass through the common bile duct, which delivers bile to the intestine. Bile participates in the digestion of fat in food. When a gallstone lodges itself in the common bile duct and blocks bile flow, symptoms arise from pressure, stretching of the tissues, and even infection because there is no longer any flow. The situation causes cells in that location to fail and rupture, thus releasing a molecule called adenosine triphosphate or ATP. ATP, a source of chemical energy for the cells, exists inside all living cells in large quantities but normally remains inside intact cells. Once it spills out of a ruptured cell, it will come in contact with the membrane of specific nerve fibers, triggering a pain receptor that lets the brain know a problem exists. Having gallstones does not itself create symptoms. The gallstones only cause pain when they get large enough to block the common bile duct and rupture cells. Finding gallstones inside the gallbladder does not prove they caused discomfort for the patient, but it makes it easy to conclude that they could be the culprit.

Leslie's surgery went smoothly, and she went from the recovery room to a regular hospital room before the sun rose on Saturday morning. She received routine pain medications appropriate for post-op comfort during the day, although her nurse noted on her chart that she seemed to have much more pain than the norm. Her surgeon checked on her in person that morning and spoke to the nurse by phone about her level of discomfort in the afternoon. By early evening, Leslie had even more pain, a fast heart rate, and elevated blood pressure. Her surgeon went back to the hospital to sort out what was happening. As he arrived at the hospital, he heard an alarm sounding for the emergency resuscitation crew. Leslie's nurse called the crew because Leslie suddenly had become unresponsive. The team did everything possible, but that evening, Leslie died from a ruptured abdominal aortic aneurysm. She died from a missed diagnosis made by good people acting in good faith. In retrospect, the ultrasound examination could have picked up an aneurysm, but finding the gallstones may have caused further scrutiny to seem unnecessary. Leslie had a family history of vascular disease, but not enough to suggest she would have a life-threatening vascular problem.

What is a ruptured abdominal aortic aneurysm? The aorta is the largest artery in the human body, carrying blood from the heart to the entire body. On its journey, it travels down through the abdomen in the midline close to the spinal column. An artery contains blood under pressure created by the beating of the heart. The artery wall has connective tissue and smooth muscle layers to provide the mechanical strength necessary to contain the pressure. Occasionally, an artery has a defect that allows blood to work its way into the artery's wall. That process separates layers of the wall and forms a bulge in the wall. As time goes on, that bulge can grow and eventually burst. Bursting means that blood suddenly shoots out into the space around the artery. If the hole occurs in the abdomen, blood pours out into the potential void around those organs, leaving very little blood circulating to supply the needs of the body's tissues and organs.

Since the brain uses lots of energy, such a loss of blood volume and pressure shows up quickly as a loss of consciousness. Usually, before an aneurysm bursts, it leaks blood. The blood cells that have escaped fracture and release adenosine triphosphate, causing pain just as we described the pain from gallstones. The human body detects tissue injury without differentiating the type of tissue. A ruptured artery creates pain no different in its messaging than a blocked common bile duct. Leslie only knew she had pain in her abdomen that she felt radiated into her back.

The Federal Government reports that mistakes in medical diagnoses in America contribute causally to the death of more than 90,000 Americans annually. They define an erroneous diagnosis as a failure to identify the correct cause of a patient's disorder or a significant delay in finding that cause. The size of this problem may represent new information for many Americans. No one seems eager to ensure everyone knows how often patients receive an incorrect medical diagnosis. We commonly can hear a diagnostic snafu story amongst guests at a cocktail party. At a mistake rate of one in seven, almost everyone might experience such an event in their lifetime. Most such errors are not serious problems. Leslie was unlucky enough to experience a diagnostic mistake that ended her life. A recent paper in the medical literature reported that in one hospital survey, as many as 60% of abdominal aortic aneurysms, because of their variable symptoms, were initially misdiagnosed.

Mistakes in diagnosis can and do happen to a vast array of patients. Singer Lady Gaga was pronounced to have muscle strain in 2012, but she had broken her hip, a problem that required surgical treatment and cancellation of her concert tour that year. Actor Woody Harrelson was found to have testicular cancer in 1987, but it was really pancreatitis. Michael Jackson was treated for vitiligo in 1986, but he had a more systemic illness called lupus. Journalist Tom Brokaw was reportedly treated for back pain for a significant period before doctors discovered he had a cancer of the blood that invades bone marrow called multiple myeloma.

Physicians also make mistakes when their patients are not celebrities.

It would be nice if we could give you a list of the common problems that get misdiagnosed so everyone could interrogate their physician intensely if they suggest you have something on the list. Unfortunately, there is no such list. The problem is not limited to a few specific conditions, although the frequency of mistakes varies widely. Instead, experts tend to agree that errors primarily arise out of taking certain shortcuts in the traditional diagnostic process. Unfortunately, these shortcuts have essentially become the norm.

Experts have also noted that the error rate may be slightly higher in pediatric patients because children cannot precisely describe their symptoms. We all react more emotionally to mistakes that involve children, and indeed, outrage in such cases appears to invoke many of the efforts in society to reduce such errors. We will discuss these later in the book.

You might feel exempt from ever experiencing any harm from a missed diagnosis. Most people have complete faith in, even admiration for, their primary medical care provider. Indeed, medical schools carefully select each student for admission into the arduous training required to practice all of the medical specialties. Indeed, you have every reason to feel confident that your chosen primary physician has nothing close to that high level of diagnostic mistakes. It must be other patients' physicians that are failing so frequently in this manner. One in seven mistakes sounds like a C-level performance, not the A+ performance we all expect.

We do not doubt the excellence of the physicians we carefully select for ourselves because they are right there when we need them. Indeed, we picked them specifically because our most trusted friends bragged to us about their dedication and attentive bedside manner. Everyone assured us that our chosen physician would minister to our every need assiduously and we found that to be true.

So, how do these much too-frequent, dangerous mistakes come about?

Dr. Larry Weed, a Professor of Medicine at the University of Vermont Medical School from 1969 to 1981, was one of the first physicians to talk publicly about the prevailing source of diagnostic medical errors. Indeed, Dr. Weed's colleagues were extremely unhappy with his honesty on this subject. Weed observed and then reported that his residents would quickly guess a diagnosis while taking a patient's medical history and performing a physical examination. Then, they would focused only on collecting information that substantiated their diagnostic guess. They appeared to settle into this mode instead of the rigorous method prescribed in their textbooks because it saved them a great deal of time and energy, and using a more rapid approach seemed a validation of their growing expertise in caring for patients.

In medical practice, all findings, whether reported by the patient, discovered by the medical provider, or found in various tests, have margins of error. A discovery, symptom, or test result may suggest a diagnosis a patient does not have. We call that a "false positive." On the other hand, if one of these falsely indicates the patient does not have a specific diagnosis that, in fact, they do have, we call that a "false negative." When a physician has guessed a diagnosis, they may find themselves hedging on the validity of a conflicting clue as being a false result, either positively or negatively wrong. Many medical practitioners refer to making an accurate diagnosis as the "art" and not the science of medical practice. But discounting contradictory findings becomes too easy when one has immediately guessed a final diagnosis. Experts in the study of logic call this tempting stray path that creates an error "conformational bias." In other words, once one jumps to a conclusion, it becomes convenient to discount the validity of evidence that does not support that conclusion. The practice of guessing a final result too early will lead one to a bias in favor of that mistaken conclusion.

Medical textbooks for well over a century have urged medical practitioners to reach a diagnosis by creating a list of all the possible causes one can imagine for that patient's condition after taking a history and performing a physical examination. We call such a list a "differential diagnosis." After making that list, the physician should devise a plan to eliminate all but one possibility. When a medical practitioner has eliminated all but one option, they have the correct diagnosis with little doubt. Unfortunately, the textbook method takes significant time and effort and seems impossible to use in the tight schedule of a busy physician's office. Adopting a "guess and substantiate" method makes the physician more efficient, and years of experience practicing medicine seem to convince physicians that they can safely take this shortcut. Physicians are not alone in falling victim to overconfidence in their abilities, but patients pay the price for such overconfidence in a medical setting, often with significant injury and hardship.

Are we sure that the high level of diagnostic errors arises solely from a failure to create a differential diagnosis? In February 2012, the National Institutes of Health Public Access published a manuscript entitled "System Related Interventions to Reduce Diagnostic Error: A Narrative Review." That publication failed to mention the demise of the differential diagnosis as the accepted path to making the correct diagnosis. Instead, this review suggested we blame clinician cognitive factors, system factors, and even patient factors for mistakes. Similar reports authored by physicians from the Agency for Healthcare Research and Quality in the same period failed to mention that hospital medical records rarely include a differential diagnosis. By contrast, in 2014, Jason Maude, not a physician, wrote an article entitled "Differential diagnosis: the key to reducing diagnosis error, measuring diagnosis and a mechanism to reduce healthcare costs." We will hear much more about Jason Maude later in this book. More recently, we find other publications showing automated differential diagnosis generators can improve the accuracy of diagnosis. Hospitals sadly do not require patient charts to include a differential diagnosis; almost no medical records currently contain a differential diagnosis.

You may recall that in decades past, America experienced a death rate from automobile accidents of about 50,000 people annually, and citizens demanded action to reduce that number. We started requiring driver education in our public schools to reduce the hazard. When we got even more serious about the problem, we demanded automobile manufacturers find ways to protect automobile passengers. We eventually got seatbelts and airbags. We also got legislation to mandate that passenger cars have the structural ability to protect passengers if the vehicle rolls over in an accident. It seems reasonable that engineering and specific tools are more effective at reducing risks and hazards than training humans to perform or avoid a particular safety-related behavior. We still offer driver education for teenagers in America, but we recognize that mainly design changes have created the reduction in highway deaths we have achieved. We did not reduce highway accidents by training drivers to be safe. Carefully conducted reviews of driver education results found that such classes were ineffective. Indeed, the reviewers discovered that "Drivers Ed" increased highway deaths in states that rewarded the students who passed the courses with licensure at a lower age limit.

When we recognize that diagnostic errors contribute significantly to the death of 90,000 Americans each year, should we be content with a decision only to use training in our efforts to reduce this death toll?

It is difficult to comprehend the death of 90,000 humans. A Boeing 747 jet aircraft can carry 366 passengers. It would take 246 Boeing 747 jet crashes each year to kill 90,000 people. No one would travel on an airline with that sort of safety record, and perhaps no one should check into a hospital knowing it is that dangerous. Should we not insist hospitals develop more effective diagnostic procedures and require practitioners to use them routinely? With the rapid growth of advanced capabilities in computer science, we are beginning to see automated diagnostic systems emerge that are easy to use, and they often can communicate with physicians in their natural language. Evidence continues to grow demonstrating these systems can save lives.

The rapidly emerging technology of artificial intelligence, in which computers learn themselves using training sets of data, has begun to add a new capability. Many of these systems can now explain to human users what factors led to the computer's decisions. Adding this capability, while not necessarily required for generating a differential diagnosis and thus reducing diagnostic mistakes, could reduce the effort required to extract patient information needed to achieve diagnostic accuracy. The ability for AI systems to communicate in natural language may also enhance the confidence of clinicians who would be using and relying on such computer-generated differential diagnosis lists.

Table of Contents

Part 1
HHS Statistics and the Gift from Larry Weed

The official Health and Human Services statistics in the United States confirm that diagnostic errors in medical care occur at about 15% across the board, meaning that roughly one in seven medical diagnoses are incorrect. An early report on this topic came from the Mayo Clinic where they found that the autopsy diagnosis in that institution differed from the diagnosis they had been treating about 15% of the time. When the Mayo Clinic reports such a finding, one tends to believe we have a problem. Similar studies at other institutions and various medical disciplines appear to reach a similar result at a consistent one-in-seven level.

You may feel shock or outrage if you have never encountered this statistic. On the other hand, your anger may not reach the level of outrage. Lacking an evil agent, we humans commonly do not mount the level of rage that leads to action. No one within the medical community is trying to put you or anyone else at risk. Indeed, good, caring, kind people are working diligently to keep patients safe and healthy. To lose 90,000 patients at one time and in one place would provoke profound outrage on the front page of every newspaper in America. But loss of life from diagnostic errors occurs diffusely in time and place. No one really notices. There is no fury. The victims are innocent but they are sick, even if the healthcare system failed to figure out exactly why. That makes outrage unlikely to ramp up. When we hear about a mistake in a diagnosis, it is usually because it was caught and corrected, and the patient involved is telling the story as a triumph over a disaster they avoided. Thus, we do not have the public outcry that other causes of similar loss of life might engender. Still, when you hear that 90,000 patient per year die in America from this single cause, you would certainly agree society should invest a great deal of time and money fixing this dire situation. It is worth reading this book to see if a solution does exist!

You may not have ever heard of Dr. Larry Weed. Larry was born in Troy, New York, in 1923. He finished medical school in 1947 and eventually became an innovator in medical practice on the faculty of the University of Vermont. He is probably best known as the inventor of the Problem Oriented Medical Record, a format now required by law in U.S. hospitals to ensure practitioners do not lose track of a single patient issue during their hospital care. Weed was an early advocate for using computers to improve information management in medical decisions in a format he invented and called "knowledge coupling." In essence, "knowledge coupling" was a potentially automated path to generating a differential diagnosis. Weed was ahead of his time, recognizing that digital computers could assist medical practitioners with error reduction. Weed recognized that the digital computer never forgot anything and consistently followed prescribed procedures without tiring or becoming distracted. That made it especially valuable in medical care.

Weed was especially vocal about physicians guessing a diagnosis and then selecting findings to support their guess instead of creating a differential diagnosis that they carefully parsed or processed to reach a final diagnosis. Medical schools consistently taught students that the diagnosis process required a differential diagnosis. But a review of hospital charts today will yield a thorough differential diagnosis list only rarely, if ever. Weed's criticism of physicians taking shortcuts that increased errors made him very unpopular with most of his physician colleagues. A YOUTUBE video (Larry Weed's 1971 Internal Medicine Grand Rounds) featuring Weed speaking at a hospital in Atlanta begins with him expressing concern that should he fall ill during his visit, he might not survive because of his unpopular criticism of common shortcuts in medical practice. Weed died in 2017, at age 93, in Vermont. Perhaps his medical colleagues did not hate him as severely as he felt they might. The several YOUTUBE videos of Larry Weed talking about medical practice are worth viewing and will certainly add to one's appreciation of the topic of this book. If we had listened to Weed more carefully, we might have saved many lives over the last 50 years.

The History of SIDM

According to the website of The Society to Improve Diagnosis in Medicine, an active focus on diagnostic errors appears to have begun about 2005, sparked by a medical conference held in Canada. By 2008, the U.S. Agency for Healthcare Research and Quality (AHRQ) had established an annual Diagnostic Error in Medicine meeting to make healthcare safer. Almost a decade earlier (November 29, 1999), the Institute of Medicine released its hallmark report entitled To Err is Human: Building a Safer Health System. That explosive account shocked America because it reported that as many as 98,000 patients per year died in American hospitals due to medical errors of various sorts, and their list of errors prominently included diagnostic mistakes. Previously, the public had never considered hospitals as being dangerous. The Institute of Medicine's report recommended that the Department of Health and Human Services create an Agency, AHRQ, to head the effort to reduce errors in hospital care. The report also called for creating reporting systems for accidental injuries and deaths, new licensing and certification procedures, and a focus on safety as a top priority for healthcare providers. And now, decades later, we have government estimates that diagnostic errors alone contribute significantly to the death of over 90,000 Americans annually. The quest for patient safety in hospitals has undoubtedly not proven successful.

The Society to Improve Diagnosis in Medicine officially established itself in 2011 to focus within the patient safety movement on paths to reduce diagnostic errors. SIDM launched its peer-reviewed journal, DIAGNOSIS, in 2014. SIDM has aggressively promoted training and research in its efforts to reduce harm from errors in diagnosis. In their own words, they advocate "research, education, policy, and quality improvement."

Highly trained and dedicated individuals created SIDM with a genuine resolve to reduce harm. Therefore, one would reasonably expect that it would be easy to find a clear statement from SIDM on the value of a differential diagnosis. Indeed, one might expect SIDM to insist that every hospital patient chart include a differential diagnosis with linked progress notes tracking the distillation of that list into a single correct diagnosis. One might expect SIDM to have a public statement supporting the development of computer-based tools to generate accurate differential diagnosis lists with calculated paths to parse those lists optimized for speed and patient safety. No such expectations of SIDM unfortunately appear valid.

Furthermore, searching for a SIDM's position on the need for automated tools for diagnostic accuracy yields no results. SIDM instead believes diagnosis is “a team effort that requires organizational skills and accountability to nurture and refine the process.” Their policies and goals lack the simplicity and clarity we find in the writings of Larry Weed. The Agency for Healthcare Research and Quality (AHRQ) appears to share the SIDM's notion that diagnostic accuracy requires critical organizational expertise to fine-tune the systems within healthcare institutions. Requiring a differential diagnosis on every chart does not appear in their recommendations for diagnostic excellence. They do not appear to condemn the common practice of guessing a diagnosis and using testing to confirm the validity of that guess. As we have learned, this approach invites confirmation bias that harms patients, but it is not a target for action by AHRQ.

SIDM does support a different error reduction practice with documented evidence of reducing errors. This practice has been dubbed "deliberate reflection." Deliberate reflection calls upon practitioners to itemize each piece of evidence that bears on their diagnosis, either agreeing or arguing against it. Writing out all of the pros and cons appears to improve one's judgment compared with reliance on a mental impression of the validity of multiple pieces of evidence. A leading differential diagnosis software system from Isabel Healthcare has automated the "deliberate reflection" procedure, and we will return to discuss that software later. Since productivity would suffer if physicians consistently employed a rigorous differential diagnosis regime, automating the differential diagnosis and deliberate reflection would be the ideal path to improve accuracy while maintaining high productivity. It becomes difficult to argue that automation tools in medical diagnosis should not become mandatory. But SIDM has stopped short of calling for automated tools to create a automated differential diagnosis with deliberate reflection to make it easier for physicians to reach an error free diagnosis.

Tools vs. Training

A comparison of diagnostic errors to the issue of automobile safety highlights the point that training works poorly to prevent mishaps compared with tools engineered (designed) to make mistakes difficult or impossible despite variations in human performance. Humans, after all, do make mistakes.

Notice the word design added into the previous paragraph. The field of industrial design has a foundational philosophy worth considering as we focus on diagnostic errors. Industrial designers say that good design puts knowledge into the world. Donald Norman originally created that terminology. He populated his classic book The Design of Everyday Things with door references. He draws his reader to recognize that people pass through many doors daily and never actively think about how to do that. We are rarely baffled over whether to push or pull the door to open it. We never need to stop to figure out where to grab the door to operate the latch. All that information is apparent when you see the door, so we do not need to remember such details to walk around a building.

Similarly, one can quickly get into a friend's automobile, one they have never driven before, and without instruction, start the engine and go. We can usually turn on the headlights without looking up the procedure in a manual. Yet, every automobile has a slightly different design. But they all seem to have design elements that guide one to the proper action demanded of the driver. Designers have built the guidance into the design.

Motorola reportedly wrote in the design specifications for their Razr Telephone that no user should ever have to consult an instruction manual. The phone's operation should be evident from the physical design of the instrument. Indeed, industrial designers call specific design parameters "affordances." They believe that humans have a precise mental capability that enables them to look at a tool with affordances and immediately know how to use it properly. We immediately know how to hold a screwdriver without being told. No one ever tries to grasp a saw by its blade while cutting a board. The physical design of the tool tells us how to hold and use it. Indeed, Donald Norman argues that we should evaluate a design of every tool or device by measuring the efficacy of its affordances, just as Motorola was demanding in its specifications for the Razr.

Does this concept from industrial design have anything to contribute to patient safety? Absolutely. In anesthesiology, practitioners occasionally injured patients because they attempted to adjust the gas mixture but mistakenly turned the wrong knob. When they recognized this as an issue, manufacturers immediately made the critical knob for oxygen dramatically different in shape and feel. They were putting information into the world. When that redesign did not completely solve the problem, they moved on to a more elaborate system that made it mechanically impossible for the anesthesia machine to dispense a gas with less than the standard 21% level of oxygen humans normally breathe. Again, they were building safety into the world so humans did not always need to think about what they should be doing.

Is it possible to force a practitioner to rule out appendicitis every time a patient has abdominal pain? Is it possible to create a physical barrier to prevent healthcare providers from sending a child home with chickenpox unless they have ruled out necrotizing fasciitis? Such a forcing function does not appear to have an apparent mechanical solution like our examples from the practice of anesthesiology. We might imagine a computer-controlled lock on the hospital door that would only open for the patient when the computer receives specific lab results, but that does not seem practical. However, an automated system that generates a differential diagnosis from the patient's data in their electronic medical record would appear to take us to a much safer place. Such a system might even force the practitioner to verify every rejected possibility on that list before certifying the patient's final diagnosis. Physicians do not look favorably on such a notion because it appears to introduce liability issues for them should they ignore a key suggestion make by the system. Society might reach a different opinion on the value of such aides. Physicians dominate the Society for Improving Diagnosis in Medicine, but perhaps it needs an equal membership of non-physicians to guide its course along better paths.

If you imagine yourself as a physician who has practiced medicine for a decade, you can appreciate that you would feel like you had seen it all. When a patient begins to relate their reason for coming to you, it would sound very much like a dozen or more stories you had heard before. It would seem silly to process that case with a complete differential diagnosis because your mind has quickly jumped to the final diagnosis. Evolution wired humans that way. So, it is easy to appreciate that such a physician might feel an automated differential diagnosis has little value and would never even review it in that circumstance. But would it not seem wise just to take a quick look? That is the hope of those who advocate for such automated systems. Such systems would not add to the physician's workload but might spark a moment's consideration that avoids a mistake.

In light of the difficulty of finding any differential diagnosis lists within patient medical records, some physicians have insisted that they routinely do create a differential diagnosis, but they create it in their head. Writing it down on the chart would take extra time with no benefit. There are upwards of 25,000 medical diagnoses one must sort through to construct that list. In the process, one must include the side effects of all the patient's medications and any other therapies underway. Conditions noted in the patient's family history also require active consideration. Creating such a thorough list without pen and paper would appear to constitute a genius-grade accomplishment of exhausting dimensions. But these physician insist they create a differential diagnosis in their head.

With the arrival of artificial intelligence with neural networks that can teach themselves how to navigate the search for a differential diagnosis from a list of signs and symptoms, we are beginning to hear from physicians who are taking advantage of this technology as a backup to their diagnostic detective work. Some are reporting the first generation of these tools using neural networks do, in fact, exhibit "ghosting" behavior. That means the system can invent a new diagnosis or claim a case with similar circumstances that never existed. Since these experimental A.I. systems are conversational, one physician asked the machine if a suspicious diagnostic possibility came from a report in the literature. And to his surprise, the system that was capable of responding in natural language admitted that it was a made-up diagnosis. Clearly, we must introduce new technology only after careful testing and verification. Still, machines that learn are poised to become valuable assets in the quest for diagnostic accuracy. After all, they work thousands of times faster than humans, never get tired or distracted, never forget a lesson learned, and never go on vacation. They also work pretty cheaply once acquired.

It would be a mistake to think we must use artificial intelligence to create a computer-based system to improve diagnostic accuracy. This point becomes important as our society becomes increasingly concerned that artificial intelligence offers enormous advances in productivity but also massive problems arising from its ability to create fake information and fraud. Until we have more experience with AI, we might not want to turn it loose in our hospitals.

It may make sense to think about automated differential diagnosis engines as analogous to using computers to identify fingerprints on behalf of law enforcement. We have been doing that for decades without AI.

If you are a police officer in a community of 26,000, no one would expect you to memorize everyone's unique fingerprints. (A population of 26,000 was selected for an obvious reason, the number of medical diagnoses possible.) Instead, fingerprints can be converted to a string of numbers using the Henry Classification

System. This method of coding fingerprints allows one to use a standard digital computer to identify possible individuals whose fingers may have left the prints found at the scene of a crime. No artificial intelligence is required. One can similarly code the characteristics or symptoms of a disease so that a standard digital computer can search for possible matches to a specific patient's symptoms and signs. Moreover, the general public can easily search the Isabel Healthcare database for possible causes of their symptoms online at no charge. The website is www.isabelhealthcare.com. Please try it for yourself. You will find it amazing.

Sadly, electronic medical records vendors in the United States have avoided including any software in their systems that suggest possible diagnoses or treatments because such software would immediately make that system into a medical device regulated by the FDA (the Food and Drug Administration). In that case, the manufacturer would need to demonstrate safety and efficacy in order to sell that system to hospitals in the United States. No one has worked out the appropriate requirements to certify such a system for sale. But if Americans insisted, there is no reason to believe the FDA could not do that. The FDA has a long history of working out similar challenges brought about by new technology and listening to manufacturers and other scientists as it creates sound policies. Americans have not asked public officials to move us in that direction.

In 2023, FDA Commissioner Robert Califf proposed a new role for that agency that would impact diagnostic errors. In 1976, Congress authorized FDA to regulate in vitro diagnostic tests as medical devices. However, the FDA elected then to exempt labs that created tests for small populations of their patients as distinct from tests manufactured for general public use. Over time, large numbers of patients utilized some of these lab-developed tests. Evidence suggests many of these tests may have design flaws and validation issues. Fixing this condition now appears appropriate, and the Commissioner cited his concern over the current high rate of diagnostic errors as a cause for his reconsideration of that exemption. He opened this issue up for public comment in 2023 and expects a revised policy to go into effect in 2024. This change would represent a significant step forward but only a minor solution compared to the more substantial number of other diagnostic mistakes that harm patients across America. This action by the FDA draws attention to their vigilance in the diagnostic error domain, and suggests that they are most capable and willing to be involved in the creation of other regulated tools to enhance diagnostic accuracy

Is the Use of Intelligent Machines Cheating?

Of course, building machines that perform tasks more reliably or accurately than humans alone can accomplish is not cheating. However, the humans who commonly diagnose patients in our healthcare system do not universally agree that we should rely on machines to do or even support such decision-making. They have and will undoubtedly continue to come up with various reasons why such assistance is not needed, but at the end of the day, if machines can save lives and reduce pain and injury, what else matters? Shame on any physicians who have not enthusiastically joined the fight to create such tools that have demonstrated efficacy in diagnostic applications.

To the credit of the American Medical Society, recently, they have made financial investments in advanced technical innovation on behalf of society through startups like Health2047 and Evidium. These new companies will exploit artificial intelligence and related technology to manage healthcare complexity better and enhance patient safety.

It might make sense for us all to thank our physicians for supporting improved safety and efficacy in American healthcare. Your remarks may be compelling if your doctor is unaware of these recent developments. Your doctor may be surprised that you are reading about and care about errors in medical diagnosis.

Barriers to the Implementation of Diagnostic Tools

We have beaten up physicians somewhat in our discussions of the need for tools to make medical diagnosis a more accurate process. There is growing recognition that training and diligence, the common paths advocated by physicians in the past, are not the most effective solutions. We have noted that the American Medical Association has invested money into developing new technology solutions.

The first barrier must be proving to everyone's satisfaction that automated diagnostic systems achieve greater accuracy without introducing any unexpected dangers. We have evidence in the medical literature that physicians, especially younger physicians, perform more accurate diagnoses using computer-generated differential diagnosis systems. Isabel Healthcare is studying outcomes for an installation of their diagnostic software in seven hospitals in and around Sao Paulo, Brazil. The results of that work after they had collected outcomes data could create worldwide enthusiasm for expanding the use of such technologies.

An important but rarely discussed aspect of computer used in healthcare needs particular scrutiny here. Computer-based information systems in hospitals have now had several decades of application as instruments to record medical treatment records, laboratory results, and medication administration details. These systems were introduced into hospital use as if the hospital were simply another office setting like thousands of other venues that use computers. However, a particular set of unique issues surfaced when using computer screens in clinical settings.

One of the first observations surrounding the clinical use of computer screens appeared to be a unique hatred from hospital staff members. They claimed that computers made their tasks more difficult, wasted time and effort, and degraded their performance in patient care. Computer applications in most other business arenas never appeared to create this hostility. Some experts suggested that medically trained individuals were not computer literate. At the same time, many noticed that medical care providers had home computers and used them efficiently and effectively, just like all other members of society.

What made computer screens and keyboards so unpopular inside hospitals? The answer appears to lie in the extremely high rate of interruptions in a clinical environment. Phones ring, beepers sound, alarms go off, and staff members interrupt one another in hospitals at an extremely high rate compared to most other venues. One rarely has five contiguous minutes to focus on a single idea while delivering patient care. But computer screens demand one's full attention to function effectively. Insufficient effort has gone into the design of computer interfaces that are interrupt-tolerant. It would be prudent to involve industrial designers in this specific task as we try to introduce more computer technology to deliver safer healthcare. The solution would require innovative graphical displays that project medical information in anatomical or physiological frames of reference that are more immediately grasped and managed than textual information delivery.

Fortunately, computers are becoming highly capable of using spoken language. The next generation of healthcare information systems could be conversational with healthcare providers. In the future, we may want the hospital information system to go on rounds and participate as a full partner in the conversation as the team interviews patients and makes decisions. Such capabilities are rapidly coming of age.

There are always unexpected barriers to change, but the potential rewards for embracing this new approach in medical diagnosis make it essential that society demand immediate action. Might we see other novel advances that improve diagnostic accuracy? Perhaps not, unless the public insists. We need to insist that every patient has a full differential diagnosis on their chart, and we need to watch for other emerging technologies that improve diagnostic speed and accuracy.

Many medical schools are introducing ultrasound imaging as a standard tool for all patient physical examinations. This technology has demonstrated improvements in diagnosis especially in emergency medicine. In the future, every physician may arrive at the bedside with an ultrasound probe instead of a stethoscope. It makes sense to make ultrasound imaging a mandated tool for every patient examination. Why listen to the heart when one can safely look at it and see its every movement? This tool makes the turbulence of a heart murmur visible so the practitioner immediately sees its magnitude and origin. We know now that ultrasound dramatically changes the outcome of cardiac arrest protocols because it quickly defines the cause of the arrest by allowing one to see ventricular wall movement. This visual image immediately defines the ideal therapy. Emergency medical technicians have begun to adopt this technology also for managing cardiopulmonary resuscitation outside the hospital. It gives them instant cues to the optimal method to restore circulation to a dying patient because they can see the precise status of the heart.

Ultrasound images can also provide better information on other body parts to rapidly focusing the search for a diagnosis onto the correct organ system. Our example of a missed diagnosis of an aortic aneurysm illustrates how an immediate ultrasound examination by the surgeon at the bedside could have saved that patient's life.

When medical practitioners insist on an automated differential diagnosis system, we might also expect that system to incorporate a dedicated staff of medical experts who constantly review and update its software. Updates could become a valuable resource for keeping practitioners abreast of the latest information on emerging diagnostic possibilities and the ideal tests to ensure accurate evaluations. We commonly rely on medical journals to keep practitioners aware of medical advancements. Still, a constantly revised differential diagnosis system could keep practitioners up-to-date in a much more timely and reliable manner. Patients could then feel confident that their care providers would be getting reminders of the latest and best information available to sort out their unique situations quickly. Who would not want that?

The Saga of Isabel Healthcare

Some would argue that children get misdiagnosed too commonly because we expect them to be healthy and we believe they will recover quickly from any illness they exhibit. Unfortunately, that is not entirely true, and a mistake in their care seems overwhelmingly tragic.

Isabel Maude's Mother took her to the family physician in the morning after a night of diarrhea, vomiting, and a fever of 104 degrees Fahrenheit. She had a rash, and chicken pox was prevalent in the community, so the physician reassured the Mom and sent them home.

Isabel's fever persisted that evening, and her rash soon covered her lower torso. The parents took her to an emergency room, where the staff focused on getting her fever down and sent her home at midnight. But Isabel kept getting sicker over the next day and night. Fortunately, the family took her back to the emergency room.

On this second visit, Isabel "crashed." A nurse was taking her blood pressure and thought the device had malfunctioned because the pressure registered so low. The staff had not recognized that Isabel was so very sick and unstable before that moment. They quickly transferred her to a better equipped hospital center. There, intensive care physicians diagnosed necrotizing fasciitis and toxic shock syndrome. Isabel required weeks of hospitalization and more than twenty surgical procedures over the next 18 years of her young life. But she survived to be a healthy adult, thankfully.

The unique aspect of Isabel Maude's story is that her parents, Jason and Charlotte Maude, quit their jobs and set to work, creating a tool they called a "system checker" to create a list of possible causes of a set of symptoms. They did this to prevent anything like what happened to their daughter from happening again. Most parents do not have the ability and imagination to do anything near that level of proactive initiative, and society owes a great deal to this family. But Jason Maude remains frustrated.

The Isabel Healthcare System Checker or self-triage tool remains available on the World Wide Web. The professional tool DDx Companion is available for clinicians, but no electronic medical record system has integrated it into its software. Several studies in the medical literature demonstrate that using the professional tool decreases diagnostic errors, but physicians must manually enter the symptoms and clues to get that benefit. Using the system with manual entry requires too much of a practitioner's diligence to permit universal use.

In 2023, the Albert Einstein Hospital in Sao Paulo, Brazil, contracted with Isabel Healthcare to use their DDX Generator software for their prestigious hospital and for six public associated hospitals. They decided that improving diagnostic accuracy represented a key objective, an initiative championed by the CEO and supported enthusiastically throughout the institution. The world awaits the results of their diagnostic accuracy data, and then perhaps we will find the rest of the world's medical systems will need to catch up with Brazil. No one expects this or any other method will instantly prevent all diagnostic errors. Still, this step could be a giant one into an era of medicine in which we harness the capabilities of new technologies to manage the complexity of diagnosis and treatment of trauma and illness. Quite likely, the Maudes are to a new era of healthcare what the Wright Brothers were to aviation.

A Closer Look at an Automated Differential Diagnosis System

As we noted previously, anyone can create an account, at no charge, on the Isabel Healthcare website and generate a differential diagnosis. Suppose we revisit the patient we thought at the start of this book to have a gallbladder attack that was indeed a rupturing aortic aneurysm. We can enter her case into the Isabel system as a female (not pregnant), 40-49 years of age, complaining of abdominal pain, tender to palpation, with nausea, and intermittent pain that radiated into her back. The Isabel response will include 30 possible causes. Some will have a Red Flag indicating a severe condition that needs urgent medical attention, and some will have a "Common" designation. Common means that the condition affects more than 50 individuals per 100,000. The user can click on each diagnosis and immediately read a description of that condition to include its cause, symptoms, and possible treatments from one of 10 authoritative sources (May Clinic, WebMD, Medline Plus, etc.) that the user elects. The website even offers the user the ability to immediately talk to a physician by linking to an agency that provides such a service at a fee.

The list of potential causes for our patient starts with gallstones and gets to abdominal aortic aneurysm as its fourth possibility. The list includes options arising from the heart, lung, kidneys, esophagus, ovaries and associated structures, urinary bladder, spinal cord, intestines, plus cancers. The complexity of ruling each potential cause in or out immediately seems daunting, and indeed, the task is daunting. Becoming an expert at medical diagnosis requires at least seven years of post-graduate education, if not more. But even such experts we now recognize pick out the wrong cause about one time out of every seven. It would be interesting to know how often the correct diagnosis fails to make the Isabel list. Since most patients currently have no such list in their medical records, we lack the data necessary to answer that question. Would anyone dare to wager that this list omits the correct diagnosis as often as one in seven? Do not make that bet!

A differential diagnosis list does not automatically ensure that practitioners correctly diagnose the patient. They must parse the list correctly, eliminating everything except the correct diagnosis. “Parse” is a term used in computer science to mean processing an input and performing specific actions to reach a desired conclusion. A mathematician would suggest that all other things being equal, the practitioner should start by selecting a test that cuts the possible diagnoses at least in half. If one had four tests that could each reduce the possible candidates by half, then thirty possible diagnoses could go to 15, then 7, then 3, then 1. Unfortunately, all diagnostic tests are not equal. Medical tests have widely divergent costs, dangers, and reliabilities. Some tests are positive for a single diagnosis, and others can be positive for multiple conditions. It might take 29 tests to reduce 30 possible diagnoses to a single accurate conclusion. Selecting a path to distill many diagnostic possibilities quickly down to one final answer can become an incredibly complex task.

If we could all agree that every patient should have a complete differential diagnosis, the next step might call for developing computer algorithms to calculate the optimal method to parse that differential diagnosis list, optimal in cost and patient safety. It makes little sense to work on that problem until we make sure patients indeed get a differential diagnosis. Remember, the Society of Improving Diagnosis in Medicine has yet to call for a differential diagnosis for every patient. Are they really content with moving forward without relying on a differential diagnosis? Do they have any evidence to suggest we no longer need that step in a highly accurate diagnostic process?

How Can Patients Speed Up Progress?

In October 2023, the Society to Improve Diagnosis in Medicine, SIDM, invited CNN Washington Anchor Jake Tapper and his daughter Alice Tapper to share their experience with a life-threatening missed medical diagnosis. At the meeting, journalist Jake Tapper pledged to continue to advocate for research into methods to make diagnostic errors vanish.

Suppose one reviews the publicly available messaging from the Society's October Meeting. They will not hear a call for requiring differential diagnosis lists on every patient chart or a plea for broader use of tools like the professional version of the Isabel Symptom Checker. Instead, SIDM talks about the need for more research to understand how mistakes happen and a greater need for patient participation in reducing such errors.

Why do we have a gap between the goals of the SIDM and the concept of automated differential diagnosis tools to make the traditional path to diagnosis rapid, robust, and accurate? The problem lies in complexity management, as Robert Wears and Kathleen Sutcliffe argue in their book Still Not Safe: Patient Safety and the Middle-Managing of American Medicine. The focus on complexity appears to invite non-physician skill sets into solving this problem. Medicine has a tradition of protective ownership of everything medical, but that stance no longer best serves society. Knowledge management has different skill sets with new and powerful gifts to bestow. The medical community needs to open itself to their help, and patients may need to rise and demand that happen.

Jason Maude and Jake Tapper have pledged to noble goals and deserve public support and recognition. Senators Bernie Sanders and Elizabeth Warren have held hearings on patient safety and continue to advocate for patients. We should thank them for their efforts and ask them to continue to work to make automated differential diagnosis software available throughout our healthcare system. We all must demand that our hospitals have a differential diagnosis on every patient chart. We understand they cannot do that alone. Still, our demands should encourage them to insist electronic medical records systems make that happen without significantly burdening medical staff productivity.

Please do not allow anyone to suggest that diagnostic errors arise from patients' inability to relate their symptoms accurately. Professionals do not blame their clients for their mistakes. Physicians are not following the steps enunciated in their own textbooks and training materials, and they need to admit that and fix that deficit with the help of information experts. To continue to claim that they need more research into the causes of mistakes insults themselves and their patients' intelligence.

The United States Congress has held at least one hearing on patient safety. It would seem appropriate to ask your representatives in Congress to give some attention to mistakes in medical diagnosis. The Affordable Care Act required hospitals to use the Problem Oriented Medical Record format. That suggests passing a law requiring hospitals to maintain a differential diagnosis list on every chart would be possible. Such a requirement would encourage the use of electronic systems to generate that list. That might involve FDA scrutiny, but the FDA has never stood in the way of progress and usually contributes considerably to the safety and reliability of the systems it regulates.

One could also write to Jake Tapper at CNN (his email address is JakeTapper@gmail.com) and ask him to use his influence to keep our nation's attention on the diagnostic error problem. Similarly, letters to thank and encourage Jason Maude at Isabel Healthcare or to Epic and Oracle/Cerner, the two significant vendors for our leading hospital information systems, would not hurt. Remember that diagnostic errors injure more Americans each year than automobile accidents have ever. Public outrage did bring about engineering improvements that make automobiles significantly safer.

How might the introduction of computer-generated differential diagnosis likely play out? Might physicians recognize the need and insist hospitals recognize that necessity? Probably not. Physicians appear entrenched in the guess-and-verify approach, and the appearance of an automated differential diagnosis list on the patient's chart would disturb their usual process. Many physicians feel the current norm has become their process for recognizing a diagnosis and then astutely selecting an economical set of steps to confirm the diagnosis they identified from their experience. They do not view the diagnosis that comes quickly to mind as a guess but instead, see that choice as the product of their knowledge gained through long hours of study and patient care. With that perspective, an independent differential diagnosis generated for the patient's chart constitutes a distraction and perhaps a liability. Both make this an unwanted step. That posture does not best serve society at large.

Practicing physicians find themselves concerned about the high rate of diagnostic errors but seem to prefer the strategy of the Society for Improving Diagnosis in Medicine. That strategy sees the problem as requiring only an extra measure of diligence, always considering what else might be the cause. and paying attention to a few common mistakes in logic. That appear to feel those steps solve the problem.

Books like this, newspaper articles about deaths from diagnostic mistakes, T.V. documentaries, and mass media might raise public awareness to a level that would force hospitals to acquire the tools we have discussed. But the lack of any clear villain in this problem makes it unlikely that the public will become outraged. Instead, we might see action brought about in the courts. If the efforts of Isabel Healthcare, for example, demonstrate that their diagnostic software now in use in Brazil makes a significant shift in accuracy for the better, medical malpractice cases might begin to focus on the fact that hospitals have not adopted proven technology to save lives. That development would appear to offer a robust advantage to the universal adoption of this technology.

Thank you for reading this short excursion into the landscape of diagnostic errors. Societal action traditionally requires societal outrage. We still hope you found Part 1 of this treatise provocatively outrageous!

PART 2

Authors are supposed to write books like this one in the third person. PART 1 abided by that rule. PART 2 will not. I want to explore a more personal aspect of this topic that could spark your interest in becoming a vocal advocate for solutions to this medical dilemma.

I, the author, went to medical school a little later in life than the norm. Before medical school, I earned a doctorate in electrical engineering, and I went to war as a member of the U.S. Army, serving as a First Lieutenant in South Vietnam.

My first two years of medical school consisted of the standard, seemingly endless barrage of lectures, eight hours per day, five days per week, all conducted in a single lecture hall that held my entire class. The first year's lecture hall was on the second floor of the medical education building, and the second year's sat in the exact same location on the third floor. We got off an hour for lunch.

I attended medical school in Richmond, Virginia. My first cousin lived in Richmond also, and she was married to Marvin Garrett, who was about eight years older than me. Marvin had risen to become a managing editor of the Richmond Times Dispatch. A managing editor, as I understood it, makes all the detailed decisions to put together a newspaper each day. The newspaper has other, more senior editors who write editorials and make more significant policy decisions.

Marvin went to work each day at about 1 PM, and his workday ended when the presses started cranking out thousands of copies of the next morning's paper.

It just so happened that Marvin dearly loved hush puppies, a fried version of cornbread. The Miller & Rhoads Tea Room, halfway between my medical school lecture hall and his office at the newspaper, served renowned hush puppies. Marvin got into a routine of inviting me to lunch every other week because it was a short walk for each of us, and checking on me gave Marvin an excuse for enjoying these epic hush puppies.

Marvin explained at one such lunch date that newspaper stories come in two distinct types. Many of them fell into the category that he called "gee-whiz." These were news items about new inventions and ideas that were exciting, straightforward, and fun to read. But the more complex news stories were different. He never had a cute name for them, but they were the more complicated stories that involved nuance and contradictions. What you read in PART 1, Marvin probably would have classified as a "gee-whiz." PART 2 will be the other type, more personal and less crisp, written in the first person.

So, you are reading a book about medical diagnosis written by a guy who set out to become a physicist back when America was starting to explore outer space. But in college, I discovered that electrical engineering might be more fun. So, I went to graduate school in engineering and eventually wrote my doctoral thesis on a medical imaging problem proposed by a cardiologist at the V.A. Hospital in Albany, New York. After focusing on a technical challenge with clinical consequences, I decided to see if anyone would let me into medical school. I still had some GI Bill money left from my military experience, so it seemed a good idea. To my surprise, one of the medical schools in my home state of Virginia gave me a chance.

In my fourth year of medical school, neurosurgeons at the school recruited me to do some electrical engineering work for them to create new ways to monitor and treat patients who had suffered severe head trauma. They soon won a federal grant to pursue that research. They invited me after graduation to work with them for two years as an engineer who had incidentally completed medical school. However, doing that work postponed my clinical residency training, so I was not ready to practice medicine. After two years with them, I found someone else to do what I had been doing. I headed into a three-year residence in anesthesiology, still at the Medical College of Virginia in Richmond.

I don't fully understand why, but I now recognize that a significant number of engineers who wander into medicine end up becoming anesthesiologists. In that specialty, one does not spend much time figuring out diagnoses. Our patients come to us with a diagnosis. We then give them an additional "disease" called anesthesia that we must cure for them to return to good health in an awake condition. One of my clinical professors in my residency frequently reminded us that when something goes wrong during an anesthetic, we should immediately undo what we just did. That only works when you are treating a disease that you created, but that is what anesthesiologists do.

My interest in reducing the rate of medical diagnostic errors most likely grew from my electrical engineering background. And perhaps that background gives me a somewhat different perspective on the problem. I have traveled along the conventional medical diagnosis path, but I have not traveled it over and over and over the way most physicians do in their careers. However, I want to touch on some of the confounding aspects of diagnostic errors and how practitioners might avoid them.

The 2019 book "Still Not Safe: Patient Safety and the Middle-Managing of American Medicine", which we mentioned earlier, concludes that physicians have played a role in derailing the effective pursuit of patient safety. How could such a thing happen? Physicians espouse themselves as the leaders in the pursuit of patient safety.

Unintended outcomes in healthcare are painful for everyone concerned. Everyone who cares for patients has experienced the agony of medical care gone amiss. I have had patients in my care not survive, and I have had to deal with the possibility that something I did or something that I failed to do caused that result. Every diagnostic error reported at the beginning of this book was traumatic not only to the patient but also to some practitioner who was trying to help. I have never met anyone in the medical community who has not experienced the distress of seeing their efforts go astray. Yet, they had to get out of bed the following day and return to the fight. These events take a heavy toll on everyone working in healthcare.

But why does it appear that the same people who fight this fight daily seem to have derailed the patient safety effort? That question has, at best, a convoluted answer. Still, we need to tackle it if we hope to do better. I do not believe physicians ever wanted to derail patient safety, but they may have made choices that favored their welfare and the welfare of institutions ahead of the best interests of the patients they serve. Humans can make such choices without fully appreciating their motives. Physicians also recognize that they need the confidence of their patients to be effective with their advice and therapy. So, in the final analysis, practitioners must ultimately support measures proven to reduce errors in all phases of healthcare delivery.

Larry Weed was critical of what he called the MDeity, a name he used for the concept of a self-serving unofficial union of physicians. This union appears to promote a notion that patients want their doctors to be sure of themselves and perhaps even overconfident. The MDeity promotes and defends that image. No physician would ever have a sign on their office wall that says, "Be aware that 15% of the diagnoses rendered here will be wrong." That would be unacceptable behavior. Furthermore, physicians ultimately will adopt anything within their power that can demonstrably reduce that 15%.

When you think about the best medical care available, the Mayo Clinic may come to mind. You may be surprised to learn that several of the early papers related to the high rate of mistakes in diagnosis came from the Mayo Clinic. I am impressed that they would dare openly to report on this problem. They have done so to reduce harm, and they have ignored the possibility that it might damage their reputation for excellence. I feel their proactive integrity enhances their reputation.

But more broadly, physicians, perhaps because of the MDeity idea, have failed to ask for help reducing diagnostic errors. Instead, they have held on doggedly to the notion that they alone can solve this problem. That is the tragedy! They are not experts in managing complexity, and they lack the skills to create novel tools in information science. Should not they open their doors to the people who have such skills?

Because I studied medicine after earning a terminal degree in electrical engineering, I naturally feel that medicine needs a significant dose of more folks with similarly divergent skill sets. I think medical schools need to recruit computer scientists, industrial designers, and experts in artificial intelligence into their classrooms. Interestingly, medical schools all require candidates to have studied organic chemistry before being admitted. Premed programs tend to stress biology and chemistry training. But to be very crass, 90,000 people are not dying each year because physicians do not know enough chemistry or biology. This unnecessary loss of life comes about because physicians do not have the expertise or inclination to build or seek, indeed even demand, tools to manage complexity. That's what it will take to turn this problem into an opportunity.

Additional Reading

The National Academies of Science published a book on improving diagnosis in 2016, but that book has a $75 price tag. It is probably not your best investment. You will be dissatisfied. One can find more current publications on this topic using your favorite internet search engine. Articles written for medical professionals may have jargon that is not immediately understandable by everyone. Still, articles in the popular press will keep one up to date with this vital issue. However, you still may find yourself dissatisfied with the caliber of the recommendations commonly proposed.

Health Affairs is a leading source of clear information on healthcare matters for public access. They provide an array of substantive papers on diagnostic errors on their website at WWW.Healthaffairs.org.

One can also get timely information from the Society for Improving Diagnosis in Medicine (SIDM) at WWW.Improvediagnosis.org.

The Health and Human Services Administration office with primary responsibility for patient safety to include mistaken diagnosis is AHRQ, and they have a website at www.ahrq.gov.

Mailing Addresses

(Should you want to express your concerns or wishes in writing.)

- Jake Tapper on CNN has publicly pledged to continue seeking means to avoid the diagnostic error that endangers the life of his daughter. He has an email address of JakeTapper@gmail.com.

- Epic Electronic Medical Record is a little hard to figure out how to contact since it is a large business with many different product lines. They list their address as 25 West Main Street, Suite 500, Madison, WI 53703

- Cerner Electronic Medical Records is similarly a complex organization owned by Oracle and now designated as Oracle Cerner, an even more extensive organization marketing computer software. WWW.cerner.com/contact will take you to a portal on the internet that may allow you to gather information on their organizational structure and even send them comments or questions.

An Additional Note

The issue of diagnostic errors has vast importance, affects millions of people, and costs society a lot of money and lost productivity. No one should dare to write about anything that crucial without plenty of help and support. I have communicated often with Jason Maude and feel privileged that he would always promptly respond and answer my questions.

I needed someone to read various drafts of this text and point out things that were unclear, misleading, or poorly expressed. Dr. Art Dimock volunteered to do that job. And he did it magnificently. Art is retired from a teaching and administrative position in the Chemistry Department at the University of Connecticut. But more than that, he is an intelligent, avuncular individual everyone enjoys being around. Years ago, he narrated a video I wrote with him entitled "Calculus with Confidence" that one can view on YouTube (https://youtu.be/a9XNg-SOIUM?si=fuS5fpVokHZOwfwh), and almost 100,000 people have watched it. The video tries to make calculus a visual concept that is easy to grasp. Art's friendly, relaxed delivery makes the video effective, and I wish I had him as a professor when I struggled through a rapid-fire organic chemistry class that tortured me during a summer school term many, many years ago. Art allowed me to get away with suggesting that organic chemistry may not represent the most essential prerequisite one needs for success in medical practice. As I said, he is very kind!

As a courtesy, we sent a draft of this book to Jason Maude at Isabel Healthcare. Previously, I had exchanged emails with Jason, and he was always prompt with a friendly answer. Sending him a book draft seemed much more burdensome. But he graciously read the draft and returned a page of comments, all of which I have tried to build into the final text. I would note that Jason objected specifically to what he called my "wildly overstated" efforts to praise his accomplishments. I expected that and made no changes. He also mentioned in his comments that a great deal more can be done to improve the systems he has played a significant role in creating, but more importantly, he added, "We are back to the same issue. Will physicians use it?"

Now that you have read this book, you share the burden of ensuring that the methods that we know will save lives become mandatory in our healthcare system. Knowledge can often become a heavy burden.

HILL GRIFFITH PULISHING

Made in the USA
Las Vegas, NV
09 July 2025

24660938R00030